Bringing
SEVENTH-DAY ADVENTISTS

to the

TEST

Spiritual Dangers

in

HEALTH CARE

by
Vernon Sparks, M.D.

Published
by

DIGITAL INSPIRATION
1481 Reagan Valley Road
Tellico Plains, TN 37385
www.vsdigitalinspiration.com

Contents

—————

1

End-Time Methods of Healing

IN a letter dated September 16, 1892, the servant of the Lord, Ellen G. White, penned some counsel from God which has special significance for those living in this last period of time:

"Perilous times are before us. The whole world will be involved in perplexity and distress, disease of every kind will be upon the human family, and such ignorance as now prevails concerning the laws of health would result in great suffering and the loss of many lives that might be saved. . . .

"As religious aggression subverts the liberties of our nation, those who would stand for freedom of conscience will be placed in unfavorable positions. For their own sake, they should, while they have opportunity, become intelligent in regard to disease, its causes, prevention, and cure. And those who do this will find a field of labor anywhere. There will be suffering ones, plenty of them, who will need help, not only among those of our own faith, but largely among those who know not the truth." *Counsels on Health,* 504, 506.

These words were written in the context of the importance of training nurses and physicians. In reality, though, these instructions from the Lord are directed to every follower of Christ. At baptism, each one of us was set apart to be educated in, and to do, Christ's medical missionary work:

"The Lord wants every one of us to educate himself for God. At baptism, in the name of the Father, and of the Son, and of the Holy Ghost we were set apart to engage in the very work that Christ came to the world to do. What was He?—In the highest sense He was a missionary, and He was a healing missionary." *Review and*

Herald, January 7, 1902.

All true believers are to be involved in meeting the physical needs of those around them:

"The Saviour lived on this earth a life that love for God will constrain every true believer in Christ to live. Following His example, in our medical missionary work we shall reveal to the world that we are His representatives, and that our credentials are from above." Ibid., June 16, 1904.

The true interpretation of the gospel is to work the way Christ worked:

"The union of Christlike work for the body and Christlike work for the soul is the true interpretation of the gospel." *My Life Today,* 224.

We are each to combine ministry to the soul with ministry for the body:

"In one hand they are to carry the gospel for the relief of sin-burdened souls, and in the other hand they are to carry remedies for the relief of physical suffering. Thus they will be true medical missionaries for God." *Medical Ministry,* 328.

False Healing as a Test

In 1904 God led the prophetess to warn His people that in finishing the work that Christ began on earth—the healing ministry—they would encounter false methodology that would severely test them. It was predicted that many will depart from the truth because of disagreements over how best to meet the needs of those who are ill:

"Wonderful scenes, with which Satan will be closely connected, will soon take place. God's Word declares that Satan will work miracles. He will make people sick, and then will suddenly remove from them his satanic power. They will then be regarded as healed. These works of apparent healing *will bring Seventh-day Adventists to the test.* Many who have had great light will fail to walk in the light, because they have not become one with Christ." *Selected Messages,* book 2, 53. (All emphasis supplied unless otherwise noted.)

Agents of Satan

We are told that Satan's crowning act of deception will be to personate Christ and His healing miracles. See *The Great Controversy*, 624. However, in 1862 God had explained that this deceptive work would be instigated by the evil angels and would thus, undoubtedly, precede Satan's personation of Christ. We are warned that Satan's evil angels will "assume new ground" with the intent to take us off guard:

"If our eyes could be opened to discern the fallen angels at work with those who feel at ease and consider themselves safe, we would not feel so secure. Evil angels are upon our track every moment. We expect a readiness on the part of bad men to act as Satan suggests; but while our minds are unguarded against his invisible agents, they assume new ground and work marvels and miracles in our sight. Are we prepared to resist them by the Word of God, the only weapon we can use successfully?

"Some will be tempted to receive these wonders as from God. The sick will be healed before us. Miracles will be performed in our sight. Are we prepared for the trial which awaits us when the lying wonders of Satan shall be more fully exhibited? Will not many souls be ensnared and taken?" *Testimonies,* vol. 1, 302.

Satan and his evil angels will work through human agents who will claim to miraculously cure disease. Their claims will appear as true miracles, but they will work by first causing the disease through satanic power and then removing it by the same power:

"Men under the influence of evil spirits will work miracles. They will make people sick by casting their spell upon them, and will then remove the spell, leading others to say that those who were sick have been miraculously healed." *Selected Messages,* book 2, 53.

Not all "healing" agents of Satan will present their work as miraculous or supernatural. Many false cures will be presented with scientific-sounding explanations. Many false methods of healing will be presented with claims that they are based upon the laws of the Creator, when, in reality, their success may be the results of the working of Satan's electric currents.

The miracles of healing that bring Seventh-day Adventists and all Christians to the test, and which will cause many to depart from the faith, may seem to be the natural outworking of simple methods of diagnosis and treatment. These false miracles may even be mixed with the eight natural remedies such as exercise, proper diet, and so on, but the end results may well cause many to lose their way. Just as the doctrinal counterfeits of Satan lie close to the path of truth, just so will error appear very much like truth in the end-time health ministry.

False Science of the Mind

We are told that as we near the close of probation Satan will work increasingly through the sciences of the mind:

"In these days when skepticism and infidelity so often appear in a scientific garb, we need to be guarded on every hand. Through this means our great adversary is deceiving thousands, and leading them captive according to his will. The advantage he takes of the sciences, sciences which pertain to the human mind, is tremendous. Here, serpentlike, he imperceptibly creeps in to corrupt the work of God.

"This entering in of Satan through the sciences is well devised. Through the channel of phrenology, psychology, and mesmerism [hypnosis], he comes more directly to the people of this generation, and works with that power which is *to characterize his efforts near the close of probation.*" *Selected Messages,* book 2, 351.

We are warned that the agents of Satan, rather than professing to use supernatural power, will tend to give credit to scientific-sounding, magnetic and electric energies, or to latent powers within the mind. In reality, they will be using Satan's electric currents to cast a spell over the souls as well as the bodies of their patients:

"The apostles of nearly all forms of spiritism claim to have power to heal. They attribute this power to electricity, magnetism, the so-called sympathetic remedies, or to latent forces within the mind of man. . . .

"Satanic agents claim to cure disease. They attribute their power to electricity, magnetism, or the so-called sympathetic remedies, while in truth they are but channels for Satan's electric currents. By this means he casts his spell over the bodies and souls of men." *Mind, Character, and Personality,* vol. 2, 701.

It will require great watchfulness to be safeguarded from deception by the false healing methods of Satan's agents. Evil spirits will cast spells upon people, causing disease. These spirits will then allow their agents to remove the spells and the diseases, resulting in cures that are considered to be miraculous:

"I am instructed to say that in the future great watchfulness will be needed. There is to be among God's people no spiritual stupidity. Evil spirits are actively engaged in seeking to control the minds of human beings. Men are binding up in bundles, ready to be consumed by the fires of the last days. Those who discard Christ and His righteousness will accept the sophistry that is flooding the world. Christians are to be sober and vigilant, steadfastly resisting their adversary the devil, who is going about as a roaring lion, seeking whom he may devour." *Selected Messages,* book 2, 53.

Natural or Supernatural

A miracle is any event or healing that is not the natural result of obedience to the laws of nature. Methods of diagnosis and treatment that are not explainable by our knowledge of anatomy, physiology, biochemistry, pathology, and so on, may be operating through the result of supernatural power. God's miracles and methods, including the biblically inspired procedure of anointing by the elders (see James 5:14), will be associated with a seeking to harmonize with the Creator's natural laws. Satan's miracles and methods will be in an atmosphere of unconcern regarding, or the ignoring of, or the disobedience of, the Creator's laws.

Methods of diagnosis and/or methods of treatment that

are not explainable by natural science, or approved by a "thus saith the Lord," may very well be used by agents of Satan to produce cures through the use of hypnosis or Satan's electric currents. This is especially true of those methods that purportedly work through magnetic or electric currents or energies, or through the "inner powers" of the mind or body. Such false methods of diagnosis and treatment are presently bringing Christians to the test, and will increasingly do so.

These false methods of healing will readily be accepted by those who do not believe in a supernatural adversary, and therefore, do not feel the need to know whether a given cure is rational—in harmony with natural law—or not. They will accept the attitude that, if a method gives good results, it is to be used without concern:

"He [Satan] fastens upon minds the delusion that there is no personal devil, and those who believe this make no effort to resist and war against that which they think does not exist. Thus poor, blind mortals finally adopt the maxim, 'Whatever is, is right.' They acknowledge no rule to measure their course." *Testimonies,* vol. 1, 295.

Rules to Detect Error

However, the followers of Christ need not be misled. God has given His people rules by which to "measure their course."

"To the law and to the testimony: if they speak not according to this word, it is because there is no light in them." Isaiah 8:20.

In addition to the Bible and the Spirit of Prophecy as tools to test for truth, God's remnant people have also been given a knowledge of natural law. A knowledge of human anatomy and physiology is essential in order for the remnant to respond appropriately to the three angels' messages to glorify the Creator. The study of physiology is to be the basis of all educational effort:

"So closely is health related to our happiness, that we cannot have the latter without the former. A practical knowledge of the science of human life is necessary in order to glorify God in our bodies. It is therefore of the highest importance that among the studies selected for childhood, physiology should occupy the first place." *Counsels on Health,* 38.

"It is well that physiology is introduced into the common schools as a branch of education. All children should study it. It should be regarded as the basis of all educational effort." *Review and Herald,* October 31, 1871.

We are told that the prevention of disease and the recovery of health is only available through obedience to the divine laws of nature:

"The laws of nature, as truly as the precepts of the Decalogue, are divine, and only in obedience to them can health be recovered or preserved." *Loma Linda Messages,* 110.

In order to help alleviate mankind's physical sufferings, and also to help His remnant people distinguish between the true and the false methods of health care, "God has permitted a flood of light to be poured upon the world in both science and art." *Patriarchs and Prophets,* 113.

To make the laws of our physical being clear, is an integral part of the third angel's message in order to prevent God's people from being misled by Satan:

"To make plain natural law, and urge the obedience of it, is the work that accompanies the third angel's message to prepare a people for the coming of the Lord." *Testimonies,* vol. 3, 161.

To those who obey God, He gives the Holy Spirit to teach them "all things," and to guide them "into all truth." John 14:26; 16:13. The Christian is to request the help of the Holy Spirit in his search for truth in the physical, as well as in the spiritual realm.

Thus the Bible, the Spirit of Prophecy, and natural law are three rules or yardsticks by which all methods of diagnosis and treatment, under the guidance of the Holy Spirit, are to be evaluated. If a method of health care is not clearly in harmony with these three rules, then it is possible for it to be one of Satan's methods, possibly working through the effects of hypnotism—the effect of mind upon mind.

Such a method of health care can be used by Satan to cast his spell upon the soul as well as upon the body.

Faith Miracles

The prophecies regarding Satan's end-time, deceptive miracles are, to some extent, already being fulfilled. There are presently a wide variety of religious faiths that are associated with purported miraculous healings.

Some of these apparently supernatural cures occur without a human intermediary. Perhaps the most famous site in the world associated with miraculous cures is that of Lourdes, France. In 1858 an apparition of the virgin Mary, on its first appearance, was purported to have instructed a poor, shepherd girl to dig in a shallow grotto. Digging with her hands, a "miracle-working" spring of water came forth. Ever since that time, bathing in the spring at this Catholic shrine has been associated with purported miraculous cures. It has been stated that there are some fifty cases a year of medically documented cures of serious disease conditions. Some cases have been so well documented scientifically that they are clearly designed to bring us to a test of our faith.[1]

There are a wide variety of methods claiming to produce miraculous cures that utilize a human intermediary. Faith healers regularly claim to miraculously heal the sick during religious services broadcast around the world on radio and television.

Christian Scientists stress total reliance on spiritual healing. They teach that all illness is an illusion, a spiritual rather than a physical problem, and thus their form of treatment consists solely of "heartfelt, yet disciplined prayer." They avoid all forms of treatment, including all medications and modern scientific health care, and even simple, home remedies such as charcoal, hydrotherapy, and massage. Since 1900 their church papers have reported over 53,000 testimonials of healing as a result of prayer alone. Longevity studies of those of this persuasion have shown, however, that it is the benefits of their "healings" that are illusory rather than the diseases. Even though

Christian Scientists do not believe in smoking or in the use of alcohol, their life expectancy has been shown to be "slightly below" equivalent, general, population groups.[2]

The above modes of healing are associated with what are claimed to be Christian beliefs, and thus are presented as the result of the working of Christ's or God's supernatural power. There is no attempt made to explain them on the basis of natural or physiological law. Other non-Christian faiths also have their miracle-working healers. Essentially, every population group in the world seems to have its miracle-working healers. Most, if not all, primitive peoples openly worship evil spirits and try to appease them as a means of preventing and/or curing disease. Psychic surgeons, associated with spirit worship, supposedly have been able to remove diseased tissues using their bare hands, without instruments and without anesthesia.

"If there arise among you a prophet, or a dreamer of dreams, and giveth thee a sign or a wonder, and the sign or the wonder come to pass, whereof he spake unto thee, saying, Let us go after other gods, which thou hast not known, and let us serve them; thou shalt not hearken unto the words of that prophet, or that dreamer of dreams: for the LORD your God proveth you, to know whether ye love the LORD your God with all your heart and with all your soul. Ye shall walk after the LORD your God, and fear him, and keep his commandments, and obey his voice, and ye shall serve him, and cleave unto him." Deuteronomy 13:1-4.

With these words, God's people are warned against deceptions that present truth or excellent results, but which are mixed with error. If all the teachings associated with the purported miracle are not "to the law and to the testimony: if they speak not according to this word, it is because there is no light in them." Isaiah 8:20. God does not and will not perform a miracle that would confirm or show approval of false doctrines and spiritual darkness:

"Be ye not unequally yoked together with unbelievers: for what fellowship hath righteousness with unrighteousness? and what communion hath light with darkness? And what concord hath Christ with Belial? or what part hath he that believeth with an infidel?" 2 Corinthians 6:14–15.

We may lessen our concern regarding this widespread, deceptive work by promising ourselves to avoid every method of treating disease that presents itself as, or claims to be, supernatural or miraculous, especially if it is associated with clearly erroneous, religious beliefs. The devil, however, is too astute to be brushed aside so readily by those who seek to hold to pure, religious beliefs.

Mind Healing Itself

While our minds are unguarded, Satan's agents come with other methods to deceive and beguile. There are a wide variety of health-promoting methods that are presented with supposedly scientific, rather than religious, explanations for how they work. There are many movements that claim health benefits from some form of meditation:

"All methods [of meditation] share certain features: In quiet surroundings, the meditator concentrates on a single point of focus—a word, shape, idea, question or, perhaps, his own breathing. Such narrowed attention compels the mind to shift from its customary busy state to one of passive receptiveness. As the mind's activity is stilled, the meditator becomes detached from thought. Some practitioners seek relaxation and a sense of well-being. Others, particularly those who practice a religion in which meditation plays a central role, aspire to mystical states."[3]

Many times the meditation is combined with natural, simple remedies such as diet, herbs, and exercise programs. One of the best-known forms of meditation is transcendental meditation which has its roots in Hinduism. This method of health care is widely promoted by health professionals as Ayurvedic medicine. Meditation therapy is based on the premise that the mind can cure the body, and it is claimed that it works by balancing various energy forces in the body. A physician-promoter of this method of health care describes it as follows:

"True healing . . . consists of a shift in consciousness in

which one ceases to identify with one's illusory physical body and instead, becomes aware of one's 'quantum mechanical body'—that energy field described as reality by Ayurveda. As a result of this shift . . . one is 'no longer bound by the concept of mortality.' "[4] Surely this is an echo of the first lie, "Ye shall not surely die." Genesis 3:4.

This form of meditation usually consists of emptying the mind of all thought except for concentration on the repetition of a secret-to-the-person word referred to as the "mantra." Such an emptying of the mind in search of supposed inner powers to heal oneself, undoubtedly permits Satan to enter, and allows him to control the results. Such meditation is described in Holy Writ as the house swept and garnished, then filled with seven spirits in addition to the original unclean one:

"When the unclean spirit is gone out of a man, he walketh through dry places, seeking rest; and finding none, he saith, I will return unto my house whence I came out. And when he cometh, he findeth it swept and garnished. Then goeth he, and taketh to him seven other spirits more wicked than himself; and they enter in, and dwell there: and the last state of that man is worse than the first." Luke 11:24–26.

In contrast to this, is the true meditation of Christianity which seeks solace, power, and healing from outside of oneself, and operates upon the principle of "by beholding we become changed."

"But we all, with open face beholding as in a glass the glory of the Lord, are changed into the same image from glory to glory, even as by the Spirit of the Lord." 2 Corinthians 3:18. By filling our minds with the goodness and love of God we are changed into the likeness of that Pattern. In contrast to the false forms of meditation, Christian meditation closes the avenues of the soul to Satan's suggestions:

"Thoughts and meditations upon the goodness of God to us would close the avenues of the soul to Satan's suggestions." *Testimonies*, vol. 4, 222.

There are many programs that utilize what is called

"visualization" or "imaging." Visualization is a form of meditation in which you concentrate on imaging that which is desired—physical health, spiritual healing, wealth, and so on. It is the concept of the power of positive thinking carried to its ultimate extreme, and it is based on the belief that the thought produces the reality. This is becoming the primary message of some so-called Christian ministries.

Some ministers are teaching their followers, and some counselors are teaching their patients, to imagine that they are having a visit with the consultant of their choice, such as the virgin Mary, or even Jesus, for the purpose of spiritual solace or physical healing. This group is reporting remarkable experiences and results. Some claim that these are merely imaginary encounters, but others claim that imagination does produce reality, and that Mary, Jesus, or whomever, did actually come to them and console or heal them. We need to remind ourselves that for millennia, witch doctors have used this same technique of "visualization" or "imaging" to place themselves in contact with the "spirit guides."[5]

We are told that we are spiritually strengthened by allowing the imagination to grasp the closing scenes of Christ's earthly life:

"It would be well to spend a thoughtful hour each day reviewing the life of Christ from the manger to Calvary. We should take it point by point and let the imagination vividly grasp each scene, especially the closing ones of His earthly life. By thus contemplating His teachings and sufferings, and the infinite sacrifice made by Him for the redemption of the race, we may strengthen our faith, quicken our love, and become more deeply imbued with the spirit which sustained our Saviour." *Testimonies*, vol. 4, 374.

However, imagination of, or meditation upon, the historical events of Christ's real life, given for our example and redemption, is totally different from the imagination dwelling upon a truly imaginary visit with Christ or with some personage known to be dead. If the reported imaging results are a real encounter with an intelligent being, it undoubtedly is an encounter with an evil spirit in the guise of the one being "imaged." The Bible does not promise that Christ will personally come to us at our beck and call. Christ's promise that He will be with us "even unto the end of the world" (Matthew 28:20) is accomplished through the work of the holy angels and of the Comforter. Christ "comes" to us and "lives in our heart" through the ministry of the angels and of the Holy Spirit. The Bible clearly teaches that "the dead know not anything" (Ecclesiastes 9:5) until resurrected by Christ, and labels as erroneous the idea of communicating with those known to be dead.

Some therapists claim that meditation is a great benefit to patients in the alleviation of stress, treatment of drug addiction, improvement in job productivity and performance, and so on. Other health providers claim to see patients with problems resulting from meditation—such as inability to sleep and a variety of psychological problems, some even severe.

Yet, in spite of these red flags of warning, many are being caught up in seeking help from the supposed inner powers of the mind. Even communistic atheism is caught up in the "research " of supernatural powers, such as transcendental meditation and mental telepathy.

Mind Healing Mind

While false forms of meditation look to the purported power of one's own mind to affect body functions, hypnosis is the working of one person's mind upon another person's mind, and thus upon the second person's body. The will of the hypnotized person is surrendered in varying degrees to the mind of the hypnotist. While hypnotized, the patient voluntarily suspends some of his or her critical reasoning faculties. Apparently, hypnosis was used in religious ceremonies in ancient Egypt. It was rediscovered and popularized by Antoine Mesmer in the 1700s, and is thus sometimes referred to as mesmerism. Hypnosis is purported to help the same type of problems as does meditation—stress, smoking, drug abuse, overweight, and so forth. However, it also finds use in more life-threatening disease conditions. In 1890, a surgeon reported doing major surgeries with hypnosis as the only anesthetic. It is estimated that ninety percent of the population can be hypnotized to some degree, and that one in four can be hypnotized so that they feel no pain during surgery.[6]

In 1958 the American Medical Association officially recognized hypnosis as an acceptable remedy. It is presently used by a large number and variety of health providers for a great array of problems. Frequently, the patient is taught self-hypnosis as a means of maintaining the "benefits" achieved.[7] Health providers warn of seeing undesirable effects from hypnosis in approximately ten percent of patients. The problems encountered included headaches, anxiety, intrusive thoughts or feelings, dizziness, memory and attention lapses—all of which may be temporary, but could last for a prolonged time.[8]

The sciences of the mind, though "good in their place" (see *Selected Messages*, book 2, 352), are readily used by Satan to lead men and women to put confidence in their own powers rather than looking to God. Satan uses these sciences to lay the foundations of spiritualism:

"Neglect of prayer leads men to rely on their own strength, and opens the door to temptation. In many cases the imagination is captivated by scientific research, and men are flattered through the consciousness of their own powers. The sciences which treat the human mind are very much exalted. They are good in their place, but they are seized upon by Satan as his powerful agents to deceive and destroy souls. His arts are accepted as from Heaven, and he thus receives the worship which suits him well. The world, which is supposed to be benefited so much by phrenology and animal magnetism, never was so corrupt as now. Through these sciences, virtue is destroyed, and the foundations of Spiritualism are laid." Ibid.❏

References:

1   "Divining Miracles: Art or Science," *Science Illustrated*, (document in author's file is undated).

2   *Journal of the American Medical Association*, September 22–29, 1989; September 19, 1990.

3   The Human Body Series, *The Brain: Mystery of Matter and Mind*, Torstar Book, Inc., 41 Madison Ave., Suite 2900, New York, NY 10010, 133.

4   *American Medical News*, July 27, 1990, 28–29.

5   *The Seduction of Christianity*, by Dave Hunt and T. A. McMahon, 160–179.

6   "What's Behind the Hocus-Pocus?" *Family Health*, February 1976, 59.

7   *Family Practice News*, May 15–31, 1989, 3, 47, 71; *Journal of the American Medical Association*, November 28, 1990, 2681.

8   *Psychology Today*, January 1987.

2

"Miracles" Masquerading as Science

THERE are a number of health care methodologies that have been practiced for quite some time that have, at least in part, not been shown to be based upon, nor to work in harmony with, natural law. Although they are frequently presented in a scientific-like setting, and those utilizing them give scientific-sounding explanations for how the remedies work, still a number of these methodologies have not been shown to be explainable by the basic sciences of anatomy, physiology, physics, chemistry, biochemistry, pathology, and so forth. Thus, these remedies are very possibly operating on the basis of mind-cure ("innate" powers of the mind), which is a form of self-hypnosis, or they operate on the basis of regular hypnosis and/or Satan's electric currents. Apparently not operating on the basis of natural laws, the results of these and other similar methodologies qualify as "miracles"—the working of supernatural powers.

Biofeedback

Biofeedback is based on the concept that we can learn to modify or control bodily responses which normally function automatically without even our awareness. These include such functions as the heart rate, blood pressure, muscle tension, temperature control of extremities, bowel activity, brain wave activity, and many others. It is presented as a generally harmless way of controlling or curing a wide variety of health problems such as menstrual cramps, spastic bowel syndrome, tension and migraine headaches, blood pressure and circulation problems, epilepsy, and so on. It is claimed to consist of learning to trust one's own internal control, and is portrayed as helping to fulfill the desirable goal of taking responsibility for one's own health.

Electronic monitoring equipment is used to show the patients some of their bodily functions. They are instructed to attempt to regulate their ongoing body activities that they see portrayed on the monitor screen and/or hear over the speakers. Over a period of time, and with coaching from the therapist, some 80 to 90 percent of adults of all ages can learn to modify at least one or more of their normally subconscious, bodily functions. This method is also used with children.

Many feel that biofeedback is generally beneficial, but it is noted that some psychiatric problems can be made worse by it, just as with hypnosis. There are other parallels between biofeedback, hypnosis, transcendental meditation, and yoga. They all are accomplished by relaxation while focusing the mind on repetitive sights, sounds or thoughts.

Buddhist monks and Indian yogas have demonstrated for centuries that a meditative trance can control body functions such as heart rate, pain perception, muscle tension, body temperature and so on. The same is accomplished through biofeedback. With reason, biofeedback is sometimes referred to as electronic Yoga or western Yoga.

Hypnosis also can be used to control involuntary processes not normally subject to conscious control such as pain perception, heart beat, breathing, digestion, and glandular activity.[1]

It is acknowledged that the electronic equipment is merely a teaching aid, and that it becomes unnecessary once the person learns "internal feedback."[2] The conclusion seems inescapable that biofeedback is a scientifically disguised form of self-hypnosis and/or transcendental meditation based on the devil's deception that health depends upon utilizing "latent forces within the mind of man." *Mind, Character, and Personality*, vol. 2, 701.

Homeopathy

Homeopathy began in the 1800s and is based on the concept that disease should be treated with medications, herbal or otherwise, that echo or increase the symptoms of the disease, but that are given in such diluted preparations that some doses cannot possibly have even one molecule of the active ingredient. The extreme dilution of the medication undoubtedly explains why the homeopathic medicines do not make the symptoms of the disease being treated more severe. It also largely explains why there are few unfavorable, chemical side effects from their medications. It is proposed that "like heals like." It is believed that the potency of the preparation is increased in a mystical way by the "succussion" or dilution process. "The power of a substance is not in the material but in its pattern. The further removed the material becomes, the greater the power of the pattern."[3] "Natrum Muriaticum," or common table salt, is prescribed at times by homeopaths according to their succussion method. However, every person knows that the more dilute the salt is in the food, the less salty it is, and thus less effective, rather than more effective.

Another example of a homeopathic preparation is one made in Germany that claims on the outside of the package:

"Aids the body in eliminating mercury from amalgam, heavy metals deposits, other toxins and alleviates associated symptoms."[4]

Each tablet of 100 milligrams is purported to contain 15 milligrams of "active ingredients." Equal parts of wild hops, bitter apple, Scotch broom, St. Mary's thistle, mistletoe, soluble *mercury*, and metallic tin and zinc make up 10 milligrams of the "active" ingredients. Equal parts of charcoal, copper acetate, and metallic gold and silver make up the remaining 5 milligrams of the "active" ingredients.

To accept the idea that to improve the elimination of mercury and other harmful metals from your body, you need to take a preparation that actually contains additional amounts of the undesirable substances, flies in the face of common sense.

These concepts are contrary to commonly experienced principles of chemistry and physics. If this aspect of homeopathy does not work because of obedience to natural law, then it may possibly have its effectiveness from the working of supernatural powers.

Reflexology and Iridology

Reflexology believes that all of the body organs are represented at specific points on the soles of the feet. Palpation and massage of these specific areas can lead to a proper diagnosis, and, by purportedly balancing the energy forces, they can cure anything from constipation to a sore throat. There are other similar systems of health care. One proposes that each organ is represented by specific points on the palms, and another that the organs are represented by specific points on the external ear. A fourth system, iridology, proposes that specific areas of the iris of the eyes reflects the health status of the many body organs. It is true that all parts of the body are interconnected by the nervous system, but anatomy and physiology have been unable to show that any point on the soles, palms, ears, or irises is any more connected or related to any one organ than it is to all other organs and tissues of the whole body. These methods claim to work through the electrical currents of the body, but they are seemingly not in harmony with the anatomy of the body's electrical system.

Kinesiology

Kinesiology teaches that certain muscles are related in a special way to specific internal organs. It is believed that the evaluation of the strength or weakness of a given muscle tells the health status of its associated organ. Again, there has been no discovery of any special anatomic or physiologic connection between any muscles and their supposedly corresponding internal organs. One practitioner of this method learned that it was his own mental state that determined the results of his patient's muscle testing, rather than the health condition of the patient.[5]

Acupuncture

Acupuncture also misrepresents the anatomy and physiology of the body's nervous system by stating that there are twelve to twenty-four vertical lines or meridians spaced around the human body. Hundreds of specific points along these meridians are believed to be connected in a special way to specific internal organs. Inserting needles in these special points can produce "analgesia" which allows for the performance of major surgery. It is also claimed that needling, massaging, or applying pressure to specific sites can treat and cure diseases of the various internal organs as well as of the musculoskeletal system:

"Acupuncturists say that health is simply a matter of tweaking into balance a mysterious life force called *qi* (pronounced chee), which is said to move through invisible meridians in the body."[6] Acupuncture is considered by some to be the most effective way of treating drug addictions—from smoking to alcoholism to heroin use. The needles used in acupuncture are hair-thin, and are inserted up to one-fourth of an inch deep into the skin. Some treatments require much deeper insertion. The needles are twirled at times to "increase" the effect. The sensation is described as "no pain" to "less than a pinprick," yet it is postulated that this nearly painless procedure applied to distant areas of the body works by stimulating the brain to release endorphins—naturally produced pain-killing chemicals. Tests of the procedure give conflicting reports as to whether acupuncture actually stimulates the release of endorphins. Even if acupuncture does release some endorphins, it is very difficult to explain how the endorphins released into the general bloodstream can produce anesthesia limited to the chest for lung surgery, and in another patient the head area for brain surgery, and during this time the patient is awake and able to drink and talk with the surgeons. The experience of science with chemicals circulating in the bloodstream to cause analgesia is that the chemicals produce anesthesia of the entire body, which is associated with unconsciousness.

The anesthesia associated with acupuncture goes contrary to the general understanding of anatomy, physiology, and biochemistry. The anesthesia of hypnosis is also unexplainable. Until science can truly show the rational basis of the anesthesia of acupuncture, we have to believe that it may very well be the result of hypnosis. Any method of health care that has been associated with paganism for several thousand years, and explains itself as balancing or releasing the energy forces of the body, should be kept at arms length until it is clearly shown to obey natural law. The devil tends to work with a mixture of truth and error, and it may possibly turn out that part of the effect of acupuncture is due to natural laws not currently known to science, and other effects may be due to hypnosis. Until that relationship can be clearly defined, it is best not to chance partaking of the tree of the knowledge of both good and evil. In spite of the fact that acupuncture may very possibly work, at least in part, through the medium of hypnosis, it is being widely used by some 9,000 practitioners in the United States, one-third of whom are physicians. Many of the results are claimed to be "nothing short of miraculous," and many expected it to be approved during 1995 by the FDA (Food and Drug Administration) of the United States government.[7]

Spine Manipulation for Organ Disease

Chiropractic claims that disease of the internal organs is caused by interference in the flow of energy to them from the nervous system. This "blockage of energy flow" is said to be caused primarily by vertebrae of the spine being "out of place," thus putting pressure on the nerves. Manipulation of the spine is purported to relieve the interference in energy flow, thus treating the diseased, internal organs.

Science has discovered that each cell in the human body produces its own energy. The electrical stimuli from the nervous system merely helps tell the cells and organs when and how hard to work—that is, the stimuli help to coordinate the activities of the cells and organs. When the internal organs are completely separated from the brain by the severing of the spinal cord, their muscle tissues and cells continue to function in essentially normal ways, thus disproving the above chiropractic concepts. The primary problems after severing the spinal cord are lack of control of bladder and bowel evacuation which is dependent upon the skeletal or external muscles which do not function at all until told to by an outside, electrical stimulus. The brain utilizes its nervous energy in helping to direct and coordinate the other organs in their activities, but it does not provide any energy for them to do those activities.

Science has shown that chiropractic manipulation relieves skeletal-muscle spasms, improves local musculoskeletal blood circulation, and increases joint motion. Thus, when used to treat musculoskeletal problems, chiropractic care has been shown to work in harmony with natural law, and is quite effective in many of these problems.

Manipulation of the spine, though, is not without risk. There have been published instances of permanent injury to the spinal cord related to this type of treatment, and thus, it is not always harmless.[8] As with any serious treatment it should be entered into only after study has shown it is indicated, and that the probability of benefit clearly outweighs the risk of harm.

Soon after the turn of the century, a Seventh-day Adventist therapist wrote in a booklet called "The Searchlight" regarding a method of treatment that related disease "to pressure and alignment problems of the spine." He apparently quoted from Ellen White's writings in a way to make it appear that Christ's methods of healing were in harmony with his. In 1911 Ellen White responded with the following words:

"Some days ago I read the booklet called 'The Searchlight.' Last night I was instructed to say to the brother who has used my name and my writings so freely in that document, that he has no right to interpret my writings as he has done, and that it is wrong to place me and my teachings before the public in the light that his booklet represents them. I forbid the use of my writings in any such way.

"Furthermore, I protest against the teachings of the 'Searchlight' as to the method of our Saviour in healing the sick. In the name of the Lord I would rebuke all such representations of our Saviour's work."[9]

As of 1993 there were some 45,000 licensed chiropractors in the United States.[10] Many of them no longer use manipulation of the spine for the treatment of the internal organs, the concept of which has not been shown to be in harmony with natural law, but seemingly more in harmony with the "magnetic healing" concepts of chiropractic's founder, D. D. Palmer.[11]

Energy Force Healing

There are a number of healing methods that attribute their success to the evaluation, manipulation, or balancing of real or purported electrical or magnetic energies. At least one system of health care seeks to maintain or restore health by balancing the good (positive) and the bad (negative) energy forces within the body, and it is referred to as the "Yin" and the "Yang."

Another system states that there is an electromagnetic energy in all living tissues radiating out from the tissues. This radiation of energy is referred to as the "aura." Certain "skilled" individuals supposedly are able to detect this aura with their hands, and can thus evaluate the health status of the tissue, be it plant or animal. "Manipulation" of the energy field is also believed to be able to treat diseased organs.

This concept of the aura also gives rise to the use of a "pendulum" to diagnose the health status of plant or animal. A suspended object on a string held over the human body is said to rotate clockwise or counter-clockwise depending on the condition of the aura. This is said to enable the "skilled" practitioner to diagnose and to treat the disease.

The concept of the aura is also used to explain how a sample of blood, urine, hair, or body secretion can be measured in one of several types of scientific-appearing machines or in a special box referred to as "Abram's box." It is claimed that the presence or absence of certain diseases can be determined by measuring the aura of the specimen.

Some health care providers believe that the touch of their hands actually provides healing power, and they relate remarkable results from this method. Other health care providers are claiming that they can evaluate conditions of health and treat disease by evaluation and manipulation of the supposed aura previously described. This method is referred to as "therapeutic touch," or TT, but the hands of the health care provider do not actually touch the patient. The hands are kept a few inches from the patient as purported evaluation and manipulation of the "energy field" takes place. This technique seems to be sweeping through hospitals and nursing schools. Some 45,000 health professionals in the United States are reported to be trained in this technique, and federal research grants are being provided to study this form of treatment.[12]

Science has shown that the electrical currents of the body do generate weak magnetic fields that extend outside of the body. The magnetic fields of the neurons of the brain are at least 1 million times weaker than the magnetic field of the earth, and require extremely sensitive equipment to detect and record.[13] Even though the earth is large, its magnetic field is weak, not even being able to attract or to create any pattern with plain metal filings. Man is unable to detect the weak magnetic field of the earth with his bare hands, yet these methods of health care claim to barehandedly evaluate and manipulate the body's magnetic fields which are at least one million times weaker! Only supernatural intervention can make such health care feasible.

Conflicting With Natural Law

There are many other methods of health care, in addition to these that we have briefly described, which fall into the same category. They claim to tap into the latent powers of the mind, or of the universe, or they claim to balance or work with the electrical energies of the body. Many times their proponents profess that the methods used are based upon natural law, but evaluation does not yet support their claims. We need to avoid all such types of remedies.

We are told that "Everything that conflicts with natural law creates a diseased condition of the soul." *Coun-*

sels on Health, 68. This is one of the reasons why God has allowed modern man to discover His laws in our bodies. He has provided us with a knowledge of anatomy, physiology, biochemistry, and so on, as tools not only to help us know how to remove disobedience of His natural laws from our lives but also to help expose the false, health care methods of Satan.

We need not get caught up with every method of health care, regardless of how glowing the reports are regarding it. Scientists are presently confused by the rapid influx of health care remedies, many of which have their roots in the mystical, spirit-worshiping religions of the East. A number of these remedies, such as therapeutic touch, transcendental meditation, and acupuncture, are reported to be associated with some degree of physiological change. Supporters use these changes to increase the acceptance of these modalities in scientific circles, but none of these findings have been demonstrated to be consistently or clearly in harmony with the laws of the Creator.

A few years ago, another health care system "several thousands of years old" was introduced to Western science. It is called Qi Gong (pronounced chee kong), which means "manipulation of vital energy." It is explained that the Qi (chee) life force must be kept at a certain level and in balance to keep sickness away. This can be accomplished by personal exercises, or it can be done for you by a Qi Gong master who performs the exercises around you without touching you. In its introduction to the Western news media, Qi Gong was demonstrated upon a Western scientist (who had been practicing self-hypnosis for a number of years and had had Qi Gong practiced upon him once before) who described the effect upon him as an 'electromagnet power inside my body.' At one point, he requested that the Qi Gong therapist decrease the energy level because he "felt ready to fly."

In 1992 scientists in Japan reported the measurement and recording of strong magnetic field energy from the hands of three individuals. The report shows tracings recording the frequency and strength of the magnetic energy force that these individuals could turn on and off at will. The recorded energy was "greater . . . by 1,000 times at least" than the magnetic field created by the body's normal, electrical currents. The reporting scientists acknowledge that they could not detect strong enough electrical currents in the bodies of the three magnetic energy emitters to produce such strong magnetic energy fields. They concluded that the source of the unusually strong magnetic fields must be "Qi"—the " 'deep force' behind our observable dimension."[14]

These reports are clearly open demonstrations of the Satan's electric currents that we have been warned about. This Qi Gong "vital force" has been studied in the laboratory, and has been demonstrated to cause physiological changes in brain potentials and in the rotation of molecules. Qi Gong has been shown to cause a sixty to eighty percent decrease in bacteria, a thirty percent reduction in cancer cells, and a fifty percent reduction in flu viruses in laboratory specimens.[15] The point is that Satan's electric currents may cause some actual physiological changes, but still not be in harmony with natural law, and certainly not approved by the Inspired Word of the Bible and the Spirit of Prophecy. Just as I mentioned with acupuncture, these other health care methodologies may also have physiological components, but depend upon hypnosis for part of their effect. Prior to our accepting and endorsing them, we need to be certain that treatments originating with Eastern, mystical religions are all truth and not a mixture of both good and evil.

There are many scientists, not of our religious persuasion, who tend to reject treatment methods not shown to be in harmony with science—natural law. They are to be commended. Unfortunately, many scientists, health care providers, and laymen, unafraid of Satan, who is out to deceive and to destroy, accept and use whatever seems to work without concern as to how a given method operates:

"Those who give themselves up to the sorcery of Satan may boast of great benefit received thereby, but does this prove their course to be wise or safe? What if life should be prolonged? What if temporal gain should be secured? Will it pay in the end to disregard the will of God? All such apparent gain will prove at last an irrecoverable loss. We cannot with impunity break down a single barrier which God has erected to guard His people from Satan's power." *Testimonies*, vol. 5, 199. ❏

References:

1   The Human Body Series, *The Brain: Mystery of Matter and Mind*, Torstar Book, Inc., 41 Madison Ave., Suite 2900, New York, NY 10010, 134.

2   Carnahan Jr., Clarence E., "Biofeedback," *Alumni Journal, School of Medicine of Loma Linda University*, November–December 1995, 14.

3   *A Visual Encyclopedia of Unconventional Medicine,* Ann Hill, 23. As quoted in *Mystical Medicine,* Warren Peters, MD, 62.

4   Product carton is in the author's files.

5   Warren Peters, op. cit., 48.

6   "Medicine's Latest Miracle," *Hippocrates*, January 1995, 53–63.

7   Ibid.

8   "Complications of Chiropractic Treatment for Back Pain," *Postgraduate Medicine*, May 15, 1988, 57–58.

9   Letter 108, 1911. As quoted in "Natural Remedies and Health Care Assistance," Albert S. Whiting, *Ministry,* April, 1989, 24–25.

10   "The Healing Profession on an Alternative," *Medical World News*, April 1993, 54.

11   *Mystical Medicine*, 64.

12   "A No Touch Therapy," *Time*, November 21, 1994, 88–89.

13   J. Vieth, "Magnetoencephalography, a New Function Diagnostic Method," *Elektroenzephalogr Verwandte Geb*, 1984, June 15, 111–118.

14   *Acupuncture and Electro-Therapeutics Resume, International Journal*, vol. 17, 1992, 75–94.

15   "Life-Force Medicine," *Medical Tribune*, February 5, 1986, 3, 19.

3

Magnetism, Electricity, and Health Reform

I N 1869 Ellen White spoke of "the electric currents in the nervous system." *Testimonies,* vol. 2, 347. This was not confirmed by science until around the turn of the century.[1] During this present century science has proved without a doubt that electric currents stimulate the muscles to contract; as well as to allow the nervous system to receive the numerous stimuli from within and without the body, and to serve as the master controller of the body's functions. A number of purported, health care methods claim that much of our disease is the result of a malfunction of the electrical or magnetic currents of the body. Science, to the contrary, is finding that human disease is largely explainable on the molecular or chemical level. A correct understanding of the role of the electrical and magnetic energies of the body is helpful in evaluating between true and false methods of health care.

Ever since the discovery of lodestones—naturally magnetized rocks—well over 2,000 years ago, man has been intrigued by the possible relationship between the health of the human body and magnetism and electricity.[2] A knowledge of what science has discovered over the centuries regarding the amazing details of how the body is constructed and how it operates can help protect us against Satan's false methods of healing.

The Building Blocks of Matter

All natural matter known to man is formed from 92 different elements called atoms, such as oxygen, carbon, iron, magnesium, hydrogen, uranium, and so on. Different atoms in varying numbers are united to form the estimated 7 million different compounds or molecules—such as the starches, cellulose, proteins, metals, vitamins, and so on.[3]

Continued research over the years has shown that all of the 92 different atoms consist of a small central mass called the nucleus, and is surrounded by orbiting electrical charges called electrons. Every atom of each element has a distinctive number of positive electrical charges in the nucleus which are electrically neutralized by an equal number of negatively charged orbiting electrons. Even though each atom is electrically neutral, for other reasons, the different elements vary in a willingness to give away or to take up electrons from the other elements. Iron tends to give away two outer orbiting electrons, leaving the atom with a net electrical charge of plus two. Chlorine tends to take on an extra electron, giving it a net charge of minus one. When atoms have extra or fewer electrons, they are called ions or free radicals, and with their positive or negative charges they are said to be in the ionized state. The opposing positive and negative charges of the different ions actually attract each other, causing the ions to tend to combine with other atoms or molecules to form even larger molecules. If a large molecule has extra or fewer electrons, it also is ionized and tends to unite with other atoms or molecules to become even larger molecules or to break apart into smaller molecules.

Each addition of, or subtraction of, atoms from a molecule creates a different substance usually with markedly different characteristics. Thus reactions between ionized atoms and molecules in the human body can form normal and thus beneficial molecules, or they can form abnormal and thus harmful molecules.

Cellular Energy

Each cell of the human body has to produce its own energy. Each cell accomplishes this by the "combustion" of blood sugar, and to a lesser extent, the fatty acids and the amino acids. With the use of enzymes—specialized protein molecules—the fuel molecules are separated atom by atom, releasing energy that originated from the sun and was placed there by the process of photosynthesis in the plants. The waste products of this cellular metabolism consists of carbon and hydrogen atoms, heat, and also electrons. Oxygen plays its essential role in the body by combining with the excess electrons and excess atoms of hydrogen and carbon to form carbon dioxide and water which then can be eliminated from the body as needed. A lack of oxygen for just a few minutes allows a harmful and even fatal buildup of waste molecules.

Ion Currents of the Body

Science understands the electrical currents of the human body to form and function in the following manner: Certain positive ions tend to gather on the outside surfaces of nerve and muscle cell walls; the inside surfaces tend to have negative ions. Thus there is a weak electrical difference between the two surfaces. With a proper stimulus the positive ions move inside the cell leaving the outside comparatively negative. This causes a wave of membrane instability and positive ion entrance to travel the length of the nerve or muscle cell. When the impulse arrives at the end of the nerve fiber a specific chemical called a neurotransmitter is released and crosses the narrow synaptic gap to the next nerve fiber, muscle, or gland, stimulating them in turn to act. It is important to note that the "electric current" of the body consists of the movement of ionized atoms crossing a membrane. It does not consist of the flow or movement of separate electrons. Also, there is no energy passed from a nerve cell to another body cell. As previously described, each cell has to produce its own energy. The stimulus of the nervous system merely tells the cell which is stimulated when and how hard to work. The nervous system does use up energy to aid the body in its activities such as digestion. The nerve cells utilize their own energy as they direct the timing and vigor of the various digestive processes. Each digestive cell, in turn uses its own energy to carry on its own work in response to the direction of the nervous system.

Physical Electricity

The energy that we call electricity that moves through metal wires to light and to heat our buildings, and that controls and powers our modern technology, is somewhat different from the electric currents of our bodies. The energy that manifests itself as static electricity and lightening, as well as the energy from our batteries, alternators, generators, and electrical outlets, consists of free, negatively charged electrons, rather than the ionized atoms that form the electrical charges of our nerves and muscles.

As we have noted, each cell is busily getting rid of waste electrons from their individual energy production, and it would not be expected for them to be benefited by extra electrons from an outside energy source, be it alternating or direct current. Extra electrons can ionize atoms and molecules that should not be ionized. Abnormal free radicals are atoms or molecules with an abnormal number of electrons. They can increase our risk of cancer, of aging, the rate of arteriosclerosis, and possibly of many other diseases.

Electricity and the Body

The negative pole of a direct current generating device connected to human tissue tends to ionize water and chloride to form oxygen gas, hydrogen atoms, chlorine gas and even additional free electrons. The latter, three substances are toxic and if concentrated enough, destroy tissue. This is the basis of electric cauterization to destroy tissue or to control bleeding during surgery.[4] Another health problem that warrants the application of electricity to the body is when the heart is in fibrillation—quivering like a bowl of Jell-O. A strong, electric current from a defibrillator causes simultaneous relaxation of all the heart cells allowing the heart to then resume effective, rhythmic, pumping action. Tests reveal varying degrees of tissue injury, but the benefits outweigh the harm.

It has been shown that broken bones tend to heal more quickly if low amperage direct current (LADC) is applied to the fracture site. There also may be increased healing of severed nerves, and other tissues, with this form of treatment. One group of investigators sought to explain its method of working: "Low amperage direct current (LADC) has been shown to perturb bone cells, which in turn promotes bone growth."[5] Perturb means "to disturb greatly." Thus the electric current works by disturbing or irritating the bone cells. Such action tends to cause inflammation with increased circulation which then increases healing. Thus, in difficult-to-heal bone fractures, the benefit from the "irritation" of electricity seems to outweigh the potential harm of the irritation.

Magnetic Energy

Magnetic energy is related to electricity. Science has shown that wherever there is a synchronous or group movement of electrons—electricity—there is the formation of a surrounding magnetic energy field. Electrons moving as a group in an electrical transmission line produce a magnetic field around the wire. The reverse also occurs. A magnetic field will cause a current to flow in a wire that moves through the magnetic field. It is through this interchange of energy between electric currents and magnetic fields that generators produce electricity; the electricity in turn rotates the shafts of motors, operating our many forms of equipment.

Human Magnetic Energy

The electric currents of our muscles and nervous system, though produced by the movement of ionized atoms rather than free electrons, also generate magnetic fields. These magnetic fields from the body are *extremely* weak, being at least one million times weaker than the magnetic field of the earth.[6] Even though the earth is very large, its magnetic field is too weak to orient any items other than other magnets which are suspended to eliminate all friction. In contrast, even small, hand magnets will orient nonmagnetized pins, nails, and so on.

Special, sensitive instruments are being developed to detect and record the magnetic currents of the body organs, especially those of the brain and heart. They are proving to be helpful in the diagnosis of disease.

Magnetic Imaging

It has been discovered that certain forms of the nuclei of our atoms such as hydrogen, carbon, sodium, and phosphorus have weak, magnetic properties. The nucleus of every atom is spinning. As the nuclei of the above atoms with magnetic properties rotate, each one produces a small magnetic field. However, these nuclei all rotate in random directions with the result that the many random-directed magnetic fields cancel each other out and thus have no group or organ magnetic field or apparent effect. It has been found that these spinning nuclei with magnetic properties respond to the energy field of a strong, external magnet and align themselves as a group with the magnet. Nuclear Magnetic Resonance Imaging (MRI for short) consists of exposing these aligned atoms to certain radio frequency waves. The aligned atoms absorb the energy of the radio frequency waves, and then re-emit it. This released energy can be measured, and, with the aid of computers, detailed pictures can be made of the various tissues and organs. This is becoming the method of choice for evaluation, not only of the physical structure, but also of the molecular function of many body tissues. When the powerful magnet is turned off, the "magnetic" atoms return to their random spinning directions.

The *temporary* aligning of the responsive nuclei by the magnetic field does not apparently affect their normal functions. There is no reported removal or addition of electrical charge. In other words, there has not been noted any ionization with its potential damage to normal molecules. The magnetic fields used in MRI do not stimulate the body's nerve or muscle impulses to act which would cause untold muscular contractions and other body reactions. Neither do they prevent the body's nerves and muscles from functioning which would cause temporary paralysis, anesthesia and unconsciousness. As presently used, MRI for diagnostic purposes seems to cause no significant effect or change, either beneficially or harmfully in the functions of these tissues.[7]

Magnetic and Electric Testing

Recently, instruments have been designed to stimulate nerve impulse transmission and muscle contraction with magnetic currents.[8] These are used to test injured nerves for ability to conduct impulses. These diagnostic tools cause no pain. The older instruments that stimulate nerve and muscle functions use electric currents and do tend to cause some pain. Certain nerve stimulators actually control chronic pain by keeping the pain nerves inactivated. Also, nerve and muscle stimulators coordinated by a computer are used to enable some cases of paralyzed people to walk.

Thus science has developed many uses for electricity and magnetism in the area of health care. These types of energy are especially useful in helping to diagnose disease. Their use in the treatment of disease, however, has not been found useful unless sufficient energy is applied to cause heating or actual stimulation of nerve or muscle impulses.

Magnets for "Health"

At present, there is a wide promotion of magnetic pads for the treatment of a multitude of diseases. "Health" magnets come in the form of rings, bracelets, belts, shoe inserts, pads of various shapes, and pads inserted in mattresses. Marvelous claims are made for their use. Up to 80–90 percent of a variety of illnesses are claimed to be benefited within as little as ten minutes. It is stated that double-blind studies confirm these results. Terms such as "amazing," "dramatic," and "miraculous" are used when describing the results. Others say that these devices have been studied on numerous occasions, but that there has been no evidence of benefit.[9]

Magnetic Deficiencies?

Some promoters theorize that these low-dosage magnets work by creating new, electrical currents in the tissues, causing some heat production that dilates the blood vessels resulting in improved circulation. Some theorize that they decrease pain by interfering with nerve transmission. Some are promoting the belief that the magnetic field of the earth is diminished resulting in a "magnetic deficiency syndrome." They claim that the magnetic therapy works because it replenishes the "magnetic deficiency" that we all suffer from. They talk of balancing the body's energies, and of bringing all of the acupuncture meridians into functional harmony with just a few minutes of treatment with therapeutic magnets.

These supporters of the "magnetic deficiency syndrome" acknowledge that science cannot explain why some localities have escaped the general weakening of the earth's magnetic field. "Interestingly, certain locales on Earth have inexplicably retained the strength of their magnetic fields. Among them, areas near Sedona, Arizona, and Lourdes, France, are destinations to which countless persons travel annually to experience feelings of well-being and to seek healing." [10] The above locations are world famous as centers for New Age philosophies, treatments, and "miracle cures" respectively.

Any film or sheet that blocks the normal, constant evaporation of water from the skin will cause a local heat buildup with increased blood flow, diminished pain and swelling, and improved healing. This can be accomplished with Saran wrap, other types of plastic, or poultices. This same effect will be caused by a magnetic sheet or pad that blocks evaporation, but this in no way indicates with certainty that there is an effect from the magnetism itself.

In the last few years there have been word-of-mouth reports, as well as articles in the scientific journals, of treatments with weak, external magnets resulting in remarkable and prompt benefit of certain nervous system diseases such as epilepsy, multiple sclerosis, depression, and so forth. In the case of multiple sclerosis, it is theorized that the magnetic field is affecting the release of hormones from the pineal gland, thus alleviating symptoms.[11]

Purifying the Air

It has been stated that lightning tends to purify the air. It has been shown that negative ions from lightning or man-made ion generators tend to cause the particulate matter suspended in the air to settle out, thus giving cleaner air. Some claim that breathing in negative ions also has benefits to the body by helping to "electrify" it. Such claims are doubtful. Clearly, breathing air free from particulate matter is desirable, especially for those suffering from respiratory problems and allergies. However, the negative ions themselves may not be helpful to the body. Negatively charged free radicals of the wrong type or in the wrong place are harmful. A good example is that of ozone as a pollutant in the air we breathe.

Inspiration has stated the following:

"You have not had a liberal supply of air. Brother I. has labored in his store, closely applying himself to his business and allowing himself but a limited amount of air and exercise. His circulation is depressed. He breathes only from the top of his lungs. It is seldom that he exercises the abdominal muscles in the act of breathing. Stomach, liver, lungs, and brain are suffering for the want of deep, full inspirations of air, which would electrify the blood and impart to it a bright, lively color, and which alone can keep it pure and give tone and vigor to every part of the living machinery." *Testimonies,* vol. 2, 67–68.

"Especially do I appeal to Brother C. to change his course of life. He cannot exercise as others in the office can. Indoor, sedentary employment is preparing him for a sudden breakdown. He cannot always do as he has done. He must spend more time in the open air, having periods of light labor of some special nature, or exercise of a pleasant, recreative character. Such confinement as he has imposed upon himself would break down the constitution of the strongest animal. It is cruel, it is wicked, a sin against himself, against which I raise my voice in warning. Brother C., more of your time must be spent in the open air, in riding or in pleasant exercise, or you must die. . . . His blood flows sluggishly through his veins for want of the vivifying air of heaven. He has done well his part in the work at the office, but still he has needed the electrifying influence of pure air and sunlight out of doors to make his work still more spiritual and enlivening." Ibid., vol. 1, 516–517.

Some feel that these references mean that the breathing of pure air provides beneficial, physical electricity to the body. The invigorating, stimulating effect of increased oxygen and diminished carbon dioxide in the blood of one breathing deeply of pure, outdoor air could be what Sister White meant by "electrifying." There is no reliable evidence that the body needs outside assistance to ionize atoms or molecules, just as there is no clear evidence that the body ever has a shortage of free electrons.

Ellen White's Use of Electricity

It is of interest that Ellen White used direct current electricity in the treatment of certain health problems. Two instances are recorded in which she assisted in the application of DC current from batteries. The first account is recorded in the *Review and Herald,* February 20, 1866. A physician was called in to apply electricity to James White during the early stages of a stroke:

"My husband slept but little, and would not be prevailed upon to rest the next day. He thought his business required his presence at the office. Night found him exhausted. His sleep was broken and unrefreshing, yet we rose in the morning at 5 o'clock to take our usual walk before breakfast. We stepped into Brother Lunt's garden, and while my husband attempted to open an ear of corn I heard a strange noise, and looking up saw his face flushed, and his right arm hanging helpless at his side. His attempt to raise his right arm was ineffectual—the muscles refused to obey the will.

"I helped him into the house, but he could not speak to me until in the house he indistinctly uttered, 'Pray, pray.' We dropped upon our knees and cried to God who had ever been to us a present help in time of trouble. He soon uttered words of praise and gratitude to God, that he could use his arm. His hand was partially restored, but not fully.

We sent for an electric battery, but none of us had experience sufficient to apply electricity in this critical case. A proposition was made to have the owner of the battery called to apply it. The physician came and applied the battery. We were trying to exercise faith in God. We called in a few who had faith, and our earnest petitions ascended to Heaven for help from above. The rich blessing of Heaven came frequently upon us all. Still there seemed to be a drawback to our faith—the physician applying the battery. We prayerfully considered the matter, and when he next came, told him we should no longer need his services. After this we felt no hindrance to our faith."

In 1903 Ellen White expressed gratefulness for the benefits of the use of a battery in the treatment of sickness. She describes its use in the treatment of lumbago:

"Our electric battery, which has been out of repair, is now in working order; and what relief it brings in sickness! Just as the prunes were ready to pick, Brother James was seized with an attack of what he calls lumbago. He had severe pains in his back, and could neither stand straight, nor bend down far enough to unlace his shoes. Sara gave him electricity, Sister James helping where she could. But Sister James was afraid of the battery, and would not touch the sponges. At first Brother James could hardly endure the application of the electricity, but Sara persevered, and wonderful relief came to him. He now thinks that electricity is a marvelous remedy. After the first application, he was able to walk straighter than he had been able to for days, and he continued to improve. Sara has given him electricity three times a day, and he has been able to keep at his work." *Manuscript Releases*, vol. 7, 118.

Thus the Lord led, or allowed, Ellen White to use physical electricity in the treatment of disease. The specific cases described are both dealing with problems of the skeletal muscles. The first case consisted of an onset of muscle weakness and/or paralysis due to interruption of the nerve stimulus. The second case dealt with muscle spasm causing disabling pain. It is readily demonstrable that electricity can cause muscles to contract.

Science confirms Sister White's understanding of the effects of electricity, "to arousing the apparently be- numbed faculties to vigorous and persevering action." *Mind, Character, and Personality*, vol. 1, 198.

Also, it is well documented that after muscles contract maximally, such as after electrical stimulation, they tend to relax. This accounts for the relief of the attack of lum- bago of Sister White's farm manager by the application of the battery. These examples, however, do not lend support to the use of electricity or magnetism in the treatment of disease unless the stimulus is strong enough to directly cause nerve and/or muscle action.

Electricity, Magnetism, and Mysticism

As we have described in the previous two chapters, there are many methods of health care that purport to diagnose and/or treat disease through the electrical currents of the body or through magnetism. As noted, many of these health care methods have strong associations with mystical reli- gions, and have been vigorously supported by the New Age movement. Many New Agers are quite frank about their rejection of standard anatomy and physiology textbooks. They say that we need an alternative model, one that is based on energy rather than matter. According to them, "We are not primarily physical forms. We are primarily energy—or magnetic or whatever you like—forms around which matter adheres. Our primary nature is not physi- cal."[12] Therefore, illness is not seen by New Agers as a physical problem, but as an imbalance or deficiency of elec- trical energy. Cure thus focuses on the manipulation of, or the replenishing of, this purported energy to remove its blockages and to balance its flow.

It is true that all matter consists of energy—positively charged nuclei and negatively charged electrons. Science has historically been able to explain the various disease processes on the level of the atoms, molecules, organs, and tissues. The health care methods with their roots in spiri- tualism say that we need to explain and treat the illnesses of the body on its elemental, electrical level.

Sorting Fact From Fiction

Students of Inspiration must remind themselves that disease can be "healed" by the removal of a spell cast by Satan. See *Selected Messages*, book 2, 53. We are also warned that as the close of probation approaches Satan will work increasingly through the sciences of the mind—phrenology, psychology, and hypnotism (see Ibid., 351), but that his agents will attribute the results to "electricity, magnetism, or the so-called sympathetic remedies [inner powers of the mind]." *Mind, Character, and Personality*, vol. 2, 701.

A scientist's or physician's report that the results of a given treatment are beneficial, even in a scientific journal, does not make the treatment scientific or truthful. For God's people to accept a treatment as being in harmony with the Creator's laws, scientists must show how the electrical or magnetic energy operates in the areas of anatomy, physiology, biochemistry, and so on, to produce the results. Because of the inspired warnings, we must not merely settle for theories or hypotheses when it comes to treatments with electricity, magnetism or the tapping of the inner sources of the mind.

With prudence, we may benefit from the largely diagnostic methods provided by science through a study of the electrical and magnetic energies of the human body as they are revealed to be in harmony with natural law. However, we should avoid those methods of treatment that have not yet been shown to work in harmony with the laws of the Creator. We should especially avoid methods that claim to cure disease through the use of hypnotism, magnetism, and the inner powers of the mind.

At present, we can say that the magnetic currents of the human body are far too weak to be detected by the human hand unless aided by some supernatural power. Scientific studies regarding exposure to certain magnetic fields suggest that if they have any effect upon the body, they are possibly more harmful rather than beneficial.

Where Disease Begins

We have discussed some of the ways electricity is used to treat health problems. Yet, not one of them has been shown to work because the external electricity is providing additional electrons needed by the body, or by providing "healthy" electrons to replace "sick" electrons. Neither has science found that external currents serve to "balance" the currents of the body. Electricity is free electrons. The body has no clearly demonstrated, disease states caused by a deficiency of electrons. Disease is not caused by sickly, defective or unbalanced electrical charges. Human disease, apparently, begins at the level of atoms and molecules, and proceeds to tissues, organs, and organ systems. In special cases external electricity can have an overall beneficial effect, but we must remember that the introduction of, or the removal of, electrons from the human body tends to cause unneeded and even harmful ionization of atoms and molecules.

Health Fads and Magnets

Man's interest in the use of electricity and magnetism in the treatment of the human body has increased greatly over the last few decades. A search for a physiological explanation of acupuncture and other modalities frequently associated with Eastern religions, has fueled part of the interest. This interest seems to go in cycles. The "last resurgence was in Victorian times when devices such as the 'electromagnetic brush,' 'galvanic spectacles,' and the 'electric corset' were in fashion."[13]

After the civil war, a wide variety of magnetic therapies became available in America. The Sears Roebuck catalog listed electric health rings and magnetic boot insoles. A variety of "magnetic" salves and liniments were promoted by traveling magnetic healers. The most efficient way to restore the blood's "magnetic field" was claimed to be by the wearing of magnetic clothing. A full line of garments were available containing up to 700 individual magnets. A certain Mr. Thacher became wealthy by manufacturing such clothing. He claimed that "magnetotherapy could cure virtually all chronic diseases and that the medical establishment was engaged in a cynical as well as unethical attempt to restrict the use of this 'natural' panacea."[14]

The Roots of Hypnosis

A similar enthusiasm for magnetotherapy had occurred 100 years earlier in the eighteenth century. In 1766, a young man named Franz Anton Mesmer wrote a doctoral thesis about the effects of gravitational fields on human health. Within a few years he came forth with the suggestion that gravitational forces produced in the human body "a sort of sympathetic magnetic flux capable of profound neuropsychiatric and constitutional effects."[15] He called this process "animal magnetism." In 1775 Mesmer wrote a major, medical treatise entitled "On the Medicinal Uses of the Magnet." Mr. Mesmer became world famous as a healer of disease through the use of magnets and "animal magnetism." In 1874 the Royal French Academy of Science established a panel, including the American ambassador Benjamin Franklin, to evaluate the claims of Mr. Mesmer. A controlled set of blinded experiments were carried out. Patients were exposed alternately to a series of magnetic or sham magnetic objects. At the conclusion of the experiments the committee stated that Mr. Mesmer's claim that the human body responds in a health-restoring way to magnets was false, and that the claimed health benefits resided entirely within the mind of the patient, and were accomplished through the power of suggestion.[16]

In retrospect it is clear that Mesmer, in his study and use of physical magnetism, had actually discovered "psychic magnetism" or hypnosis.

Areas of Concern

Undoubtedly, this topic of electricity, magnetism and health is difficult to fully understand, and thus it lends itself to many different interpretations. In trying to come to correct conclusions, we need to ask ourselves several questions:

1. If physical magnets actually help 60 to 80 percent of

the cases of a wide variety of health problems without harmful side effects, and those benefits are so prompt and easily determined—

a. Why has the popularity or use of physical magnets waxed and waned so dramatically over the centuries?

b. Why do some double-blind studies claim that physical magnets produce beneficial results while others claim that they do not? In other words, why are the results inconsistent?

2. If physical magnets are so beneficial, so economical, so "natural," and so readily available, why did the Lord not lead or allow Ellen White to identify them as a proper method of treatment—such as in the class of charcoal, simple herbs, and electricity for the stimulation of muscles?

3. Mrs. Ellen White warns us that "the apostles of nearly all forms of spiritism claim to have power to heal. They attribute this power to electricity, magnetism, the so-called 'sympathetic remedies,' or to latent forces within the mind of man." *Prophets and Kings*, 211. Could this truly be a warning against physical magnetism as well as psychic magnetism—hypnosis? Certainly, they were both confused and mingled together by Antoine Mesmer in the 1700s. For decades the association between these two modalities had been so close that the general feeling was that magnetism was synonymous with mesmerism which was synonymous with charlatanism. This centuries-long association in the minds of people was cited by researchers in Sweden as late as 1949,[17] by others in Japan in 1967[18] and 1974,[19] and in America in 1993,[20] to be a "hindering" factor in the proper scientific evaluation of physical magnets and human health.

4. Since the effects of magnets have been investigated and debated for some 2,000 years, and proponents as well as detractors agree that science has not yet found "a biochemical transduction mechanism capable of explaining how low-energy magnetic fields interact with human tissue,"[21] is it not premature to accept the idea that the purported effects of the use of magnets is based on obedience to natural law?

5. Industrial man has learned to identify, to refine, and to concentrate many desirable substances occurring naturally in nature. Some examples are the starch in refined flours and polished rice, sugar from sugar cane and sugar beets, edible oils and fats, 60% of modern medications which are of plant origin, and so on. Experience has shown that, though there are many times, short-term, immediate benefits and they are convenient to use, there are also long-term unforeseen consequences and problems. Many times the final conclusions are that the use of such unnaturally concentrated and refined "natural" substances should only be used in a limited and well-controlled way. Many now believe that the less we use such items the better off we are. Is it not quite likely that further evaluation of physical magnetism will lead to the same type of conclusions?

6. The vast majority of our health problems consist of pain and disability caused by inflammation and swelling, of some origin, which interferes with local blood circulation producing local buildup of waste products and a shortage of nutrients and oxygen. This local interference with blood circulation is the common problem of generally all forms of infections wherever they are in the body. Local blood circulation interference is also common to all musculoskeletal problems such as strains, sprains, bruises, tendonitis, bursitis, arthritis, and so on. Persistent muscle spasms also interfere with local blood flow and thus can initiate or aggravate all of the above problems.

An intelligent application of hydrotherapy in its many forms has powerful physiological effects upon the circulation, causing improved local, as well as general, blood flow with a removal of local waste products and a fresh supply of vital oxygen and nutrients. These effects result in remarkable benefits in the vast majority of cases with the above health problems. Inspiration highly recommends the use of hydrotherapy. Health benefits derived from its use clearly honor the Creator and help to vindicate His natural laws.

In the context of the great controversy, would it be wise to replace the clearly God-ordained hydrotherapy with the unproved mechanisms of magnetism in its purported "remarkable" benefit to local circulation and relief of swelling, inflammation, and pain?

7. Since some studies have suggested an increased incidence of certain diseases such as leukemia, male breast cancer, abnormal pregnancies, and chromosomal abnormalities in adults who have increased occupational exposure to magnetic fields, is it not premature to assume that the effects of magnets on the human body are only beneficial, and that the supposedly early benefits of their use could be followed by a later onset of even worse diseases? Is not this an even greater possibility when studies have reported that children who live in homes with high exposure to magnetic fields have a 1.2 to 3 times greater risk of developing such illnesses as childhood leukemia, lymphoma, and brain tumors?[22]

Conclusions

The experience of Anton Mesmer should raise bright, red flags for students of the Spirit of Prophecy. We have been warned that there will be healers who will attribute their success to the effects of electric or magnetic currents upon the body, but will actually be using "psychic magnetism" or hypnosis and/or "Satan's electric currents." *Mind, Character, and Personality,* vol. 2, 701. We are warned not to rely merely upon experience to determine a true remedy. We are to accept only those remedies that science has shown to operate in harmony with natural law, and that are not in contradiction to Inspiration. See Chapter 4 of this book.

There is the real possibility that if we get involved in treatments involving electricity or magnetism not yet confirmed to have a physiological basis, and of which we may have been specifically warned, we may actually be dabbling in "psychic magnetism" as did Mr. Mesmer.

It would be well to answer one final question regarding the use of physical magnets in the treatment of disease. With the uncertainty in the scientific field as to how magnetism really works, and as to the benefits versus potential harm, and with the silence in Inspiration regarding its approval by God, would we not be prudent to assume that the use of magnets in the treatment of disease is a methodology that Satan can readily use to bring Christians to the test? ❏

References:

1   *Medical Science and the Spirit of Prophecy*, 38. A publication of the E.G.W. Estate.

2   Macklis, MD, Roger M. "Magnetic Healing, Quackery, and the Debate about the Health Effects of Electromagnetic Fields," *Annals of Internal Medicine*, March 1, 1993, 376–383.

3   "Chemistry," *Compton's Interactive Encyclopedia*, 1994 edition.

4   Berendson, Jaak and Simonsson, Daniel, "Electrochemical Aspects of Treatment of Tissue with Direct Current," *European Journal of Surgery*, 1994, Supplement 574, 111–115.

5   Shafer, D. M.; Rogerson, K.; Norton, L.; and Bennett, J., "The Effect of Electrical Perturbation on Osseointegration of Titanium Dental Implants: A Preliminary Study," *Journal of Oral and Maxillofacial Surgery*, September 1995, 1063–1068.

6   Vieth, J, "Magnetoencephalography, a New Function Diagnostic Method," *Elektroenzephalogr Verwandte Geb*, 1984, June 15, 111–118.

7   *An Introduction to Magnetic Resonance in Medicine*, Edited by Peter A. Rinck, Thieme Medical Publishers, Inc., New York, 1990.

8   Barker, Anthony T., "Electricity, Magnetism, and the Body: Some Uses and Abuses," *Journal of the Royal Society of Health*, April 1994, 91–97.

9   Barker, Anthony T., op. cit..

10   Hacmac, D. C., Edward A., *An Overview of Biomagnetic Therapeutics*, January 1991, 4.

11   Sandyk R, "Rapid normalization of visual evoked potentials by picoTesla range magnetic fields in chronic progressive multiple sclerosis," *International Journal of Neuroscience*, August 1994; 77 (3–4): 243–259.

12   *The Journal of Holistic Health*, 1977, 13–14.

13   Barker, Anthony T., op. cit..

14   Macklis, MD, Roger M., op. cit., 380.

15   Ibid.

16   Ibid.

17   Hansen, K. M., *Acta Med. Scand.*, 135 (6), 448–457, 1949.

18   Nakagawa, K., et al, *Japan Medical Journal*, 2065, 9–14, 1963.

19   Nakagawa, K., et al, Ibid., 2253, 22–26, 1967.

20   Macklis, MD, Roger M., op. cit., 376.

21   Ibid.

22   Ibid.; Hacmac, D. C., Edward A., op. cit.

4

God's Plan of Rational Remedies

IN chapter one we noted how God is behind the explosion of knowledge in man's understanding of natural law. In the early days of our church, the Lord instructed us to train medical missionary nurses and MD physicians to be the core of our health work. This counsel was undoubtedly given in part because of all of the differing types of health care workers; this class of workers have best kept pace with the God-ordained explosion of knowledge in natural sciences—anatomy, physiology, chemistry, biochemistry, and so on. As science is discovering how the human body is constructed and how it truly functions in health and disease, many physicians and nurses are adopting some of the principles of health that are in harmony with the revealed truth of the Spirit of Prophecy and the Scriptures. This fact is demonstrated by the increasing promotion of high-fiber diets, less animal fat in the diet, exercise for the prevention and treatment of disease, and so on.

Although our core medical missionaries were to be trained nurses and MD physicians, they were to be given the opportunity to know the very best things done by other systems of health care. After being trained in the most up-to-date system of natural science, they were then to adopt all methods of health care that were in harmony, first, with Scripture and the Spirit of Prophecy, and then with natural law. The Spirit of the Lord counseled them, "You are not justified in advocating one school [system of health care] above the others, as though it were the only one worthy of respect." *Pamphlets in the Concordance*, no. 66, 41.

We have examples of how Ellen White related to physicians and to the discoveries of science in her day. Whenever she or her family were ill and needed professional assistance, she tended to ask for help from those who were the most up-to-date in their knowledge of natural law. As advances in modern medicine were made, she related to them in a positive way. She repeatedly acknowledged the legitimate place for surgery, which is frequently associated with anesthetics. See *Selected Messages*, book 2, 284; *Manuscript Releases*, vol. 14, 269–270. She herself used and approved the use of coffee (see *Selected Messages*, book 2, 302–303) and tea (see ibid., 302), if needed, for their medicinal effects. She personally received X-ray treatments (see ibid., 303) for a skin lesion. She received and recommended smallpox vaccination. Ibid. She spoke of the potential benefit of blood transfusions. Ibid. When asked about the use of quinine to save the life of a malaria patient, she is quoted as stating, "We are expected to do the best we can." Ibid., 282. She also referred to "some simple herbs" "used intelligently" "that at times are beneficial." Ibid., 294. These, of course, act upon the human body as a medication through a physiological, chemical effect.

Ellen White stated that her occasional use of "poisonous" tea as a medicine, but never as a beverage, was in harmony with her messages from the Lord. "I do not preach one thing and practice another. I do not present to my hearers rules of life for them to follow while I make an exception in my own case." *Selected Messages*, book 2, 302.

Her example reveals that she recognized that methods of diagnosis and treatment based on obedience to natural law can be a part of Heaven's health program when they are needed and when they are available. She related to the development of modern technology in a positive way, resorting to it when it offered the best results possible under the circumstances. Her example reveals that God expects us to prevent disease by healthful living. However, if we do become ill, He wants us to do for ourselves what we can through the simple, natural remedies. If we need professional assistance, the health professional is to improve our utilization of the eight natural remedies. Yet, if improvement is not made, it is not a denial of our faith in God's miracle-working power to utilize more complex methods of diagnosis and treatment to save life and prevent disability, if these methods are based upon a knowledge of, and obedience to, His natural laws.

As Seventh-day Adventist Christians, we are accustomed to being in the minority in regard to our spiritual beliefs. We are used to standing for truth even when the majority go the other way. Thus, we seem to naturally choose the minority views, even in the areas of science. We are first to test all purported truth by measuring it by the Bible and the Spirit of Prophecy. Beliefs regarding natural law are then to be measured by the most widely accepted understanding of natural law. We may not agree with how sinful man applies much of his knowledge of the natural sciences, but we will accept the scientific understanding of the majority as to how the human body operates in health and disease unless it is contrary to a "Thus saith the Lord."

All the differing interpretations of anatomy, physiology, and pathology in the mystical, as well as the conventional, methods of health care have their supporters. All methods of health care will have at least some scientists and physicians who will propose various possible explanations as to how their chosen method of diagnosis and health care is in "harmony" with natural law. Many people use various systems of health care, believing that in time scientific discoveries will show that their methods are based on natural law. The only way to know whether or not a method of diagnosis and health care may be utilized in giving the third angel's message is to know that it is in harmony with the Bible, the Spirit of Prophecy, and the majority understanding of natural law, when that is not contrary to a "Thus saith the Lord." We should avoid systems of diagnosis and treatment that are not yet generally acknowledged as being in harmony with natural law. This caution will help to protect us from Satan's false systems, which are mixtures of truth and error, and can be the means of Satan casting his spell upon the soul as well as upon the body.

Experience Not Reliable

Some people will say that they have used successfully, or they have observed others use successfully, one or more methods of diagnosis and treatment not yet acknowledged as being in harmony with natural law. They accept their successful personal or observed "experience" as evidence of the truthfulness of their methods. The Spirit of Prophecy states that experience alone is not a safe guide in arriving at truth:

"Experience is said to be the best teacher. Genuine experience is indeed valuable. But habits and customs gird men and women as with iron bands, and these false habits and customs are generally justified by experience, according to the common understanding of the word. Very many have abused precious experience. They have clung to their injurious habits, which are decidedly enfeebling to physical, mental, and moral health, and when you seek to instruct them, they sanction their course by referring to their experience. But *true experience is in harmony with natural law and science.* . . .

"Genuine experience is a variety of experiments entered into carefully, with the mind freed from prejudice and uncontrolled by previously established opinions and habits; marking the results with careful solicitude, anxious to learn, improve, and reform, on every or any habit, *if that habit is not in harmony with physical and moral law.* With some, the idea of others gainsaying that which they have learned by experience seems to them to be folly, and even cruelty itself. But there are more errors received, and firmly retained, under the false idea of experience, than from any other cause; for this reason, that which is generally termed experience is no experience at all, because there has never been a fair trial by actual experiment and thorough investigation, with a knowledge of the principle involved in the action. . . .

"*Genuine experience is in harmony with the unchangeable principles of nature.* Superstition, caused by diseased imagination, is frequently in conflict with science and principle. And yet the unanswerable argument is urged,

'I must be correct, for this is my experience.'" *Health Reformer*, 78–79.

There are several reasons why personal experience is not a reliable method of determining truth in the health area. One is the placebo effect. It has been shown repeatedly that if one believes in a method of treatment, sixty to seventy percent of the time he will feel benefited by that treatment. Also, if one does not have faith in a given treatment, he will feel that he is worse sixty to seventy percent of the time after receiving that treatment. Another confounding factor is that most illnesses get better regardless of the treatment given. A third confusing factor is that usually more than one treatment is given at a time— such as a change in diet, rest, increased fluids, poultices, herbs, or medication. Thus, without controlled studies it is almost impossible to determine whether or not a given treatment is beneficial, neutral, or counterproductive— for the patient recovers in spite of the treatments. If we are using methods of health care that we know are in harmony with divine revelation and natural law, then we can thank God for the results and not be overly concerned about determining which remedy had which effect. It is too easy to give excess credit to the remedy and not enough to God who has worked through His natural means to bring about the healing.

Divine Guidance

Because of the Spirit of Prophecy, we as Seventh-day Adventists have a tremendous advantage over the world in knowing beneficial and true methods of health care. We are told that after proper instruction in healthful living has been given, "If the sick and suffering will do only as well as they know in regard to living out the principles of health reform perseveringly, then they will in nine cases out of ten recover from their ailments." *Medical Ministry*, 224. Thus, the true remedies of "pure air, sunlight, abstemiousness, rest, exercise, proper diet, the use of water, trust in divine power" (*Ministry of Healing*, 127), along with perhaps charcoal, poultices, massage, simple manipulation, and simple herbs applied in intelligent and rational ways, will get us over the vast majority of our illnesses. The above reference from *Medical Ministry*, 224, also tells us that there will always be a small percentage of illnesses that will not be cured by the simple remedies.

Some of the above ten percent who are not cured by the simple remedies will respond to the more complex methods of treatment. The methods chosen should be the most widely acknowledged as being rational remedies—that is, in harmony with natural law and divine revelation.

Writing in the *Review and Herald* of October 11, 1898, Mrs. E. G. White quoted the following report of Elder H. C. Lacey regarding the nurses' training at the Avondale School: "In connection with the other work undertaken by our school, there has been organized this year a special department of physiology and hygiene. This department offers to the student the means of acquiring a practical knowledge of the workings of the wonderful mechanism of the human body, and furnishes an opportunity of becoming acquainted with the most approved methods in the rational treatment of disease. The study of anatomy, the form and structure of the body; of physiology, the use and functions of the various organs; and of hygiene, the laws that underlie their healthful activities, is pursued from a Biblical and scientific point of view.

"The object we have before us is the qualifying of laborers to engage in the all-round work of the third angel's message."

A practice which we need to avoid is that of overusing, and thus misusing, the more complex remedies of modern technology. Rather than put forth the effort and time to restore our organs to their normal function through the simple, natural remedies readily available to all, we impatiently rush to the doctor desiring a prescription medication to give us a quick cure. This approach is not in harmony with the counsels from the Lord; neither is it in harmony with good science.

Satan first deceived Eve by getting her to believe her senses and her "experience." After perceiving no evil results from touching the fruit, she proceeded to taste of it. "It was grateful to the taste, and as she ate, she seemed to feel a vivifying power, and imagined herself entering upon a higher state of existence." *Patriarchs and Prophets*, 56. Her "experience" in opposition to a direct "Thus saith the Lord" was then used to mislead Adam into error and disobedience. See *Health Reformer*, 80. In these last days Satan is appealing, and will continue to appeal, to our senses and to our "experiences" to lead us to live and work in disobedience to truth as written by God's hand in Scripture, the Spirit of Prophecy, and the physical world. If Satan can get us to base our health message and practice on an "experience" that is contrary to a "Thus saith the Lord" in the natural world, he knows that sooner or later he will find it much easier to get us to go contrary to a "Thus saith the Lord" in other areas. Because a method of health care gives seemingly good results is not evidence that it is based upon truth and is thus safe to use. The closer we get to Satan's personation of Christ, the more crucial it becomes that we are certain that our practices and messages are in harmony with truth and that they are not a mere reflection of our "experience," or that of others.

Emphasize Rational Remedies

There are theories which are not safe for us to handle. We must base our faith upon a "Thus saith the Lord" of the Bible, the Spirit of Prophecy, and the true sciences of nature:

"Theories will be brought in that it will not be wise for us to handle. Satan is a cunning worker, and he will bring in subtle fallacies to darken and confuse the mind and root out the doctrines of salvation. . . .

"The man who makes the working of miracles the test of his faith will find that Satan can, through a species of deceptions, perform wonders that will appear to be genuine miracles. . . .

"Let not the days pass by and precious opportunities be lost of seeking the Lord with all the heart and mind and soul. If we accept not the truth in the love of it, we may be

among the number who will see the miracles wrought by
Satan in these last days, and believe them. Many strange
things will appear as wonderful miracles, which should be
regarded as deceptions manufactured by the father of lies."
Selected Messages, book 2, 52–53.

The miracle-working abilities of Satan and his agents
will necessitate our emphasizing the natural remedies that
are effective because they are working through obedience
to the natural laws of Christ, the Creator, rather than the
supernatural, miracle-working power used by Christ in His
ministry on earth:

"The way in which Christ worked was to preach the
Word, and to relieve suffering by miraculous works of healing. But I am instructed that we cannot now work in this
way, for Satan will exercise his power by working miracles.
God's servants today could not work by means of miracles,
because spurious works of healing, claiming to be divine,
will be wrought.

"For this reason the Lord has marked out a way in which
His people are to carry forward a work of physical healing,
combined with the teaching of the Word. Sanitariums are
to be established, and with these institutions are to be
connected workers who will carry forward genuine medical
missionary work. Thus a guarding influence is thrown
around those who come to the sanitariums for treatment.

"This is the provision the Lord has made whereby gospel medical missionary work is to be done for many souls."
Ibid., 54.

Part of our task in the giving of the three angels' messages to every kindred, nation, tongue, and people is to
teach natural law and to encourage obedience to it. See
Counsels on Health, 21. We are to lead the people in the
application of the simple, rational, in-harmony-with-natu-
ral-law remedies. God's blessing will be upon such work,
and it will lead to supernatural results. God's end-time
miracles will be largely related to His blessing in the use
of simple, rational remedies:

"God's miracles do not always bear the outward sem-
blance of miracles. Often they are brought about in a way

which looks like the natural course of events. When we pray for the sick, we also work for them. We answer our own prayers by using the remedies within our reach. Water, wisely applied, is a most powerful remedy. As it is used intelligently, favorable results are seen. God has given us intelligence, and He desires us to make the most of His health-giving blessings. We ask that God will give bread to the hungry; we are then to act as His helping hand in relieving hunger. We are to use every blessing God has placed within our reach for the deliverance of those in danger.

"Natural means, used in accordance with God's will, bring about supernatural results. We ask for a miracle, and the Lord directs the mind to some simple remedy. We ask to be kept from the pestilence that walketh in darkness, that is stalking with such power through the world; we are then to cooperate with God, observing the laws of health and life. Having done all that we possibly can, we are to keep asking in faith for health and strength. We are to eat that food which will preserve the health of the body.

"God gives us no encouragement that He will do for us what we can do for ourselves. Natural laws are to be obeyed. We are not to fail of doing our part. God says to us, 'Work out your own salvation with fear and trembling. For it is God which worketh in you both to will and to do of his good pleasure.'" Philippians 2:12–13.

"We cannot disregard the laws of nature without disregarding the laws of God. We cannot expect the Lord to work a miracle for us while we neglect the simple remedies He has provided for our use, which aptly and opportunely applied, will bring about a miraculous result. Therefore, pray, believe, and work." *Seventh-day Adventist Bible Commentary*, vol. 7, 938–939.

Unsafe Health Care

Even though we may be benefited temporally by using health care methods unapproved by God, in the end there will be irrecoverable loss:

"Those who give themselves up to the sorcery of Satan may boast of great benefit received thereby, but does this prove their course to be wise or safe? What if life should be prolonged? What if temporal gain should be secured? Will it pay in the end to disregard the will of God? All such apparent gain will prove at last an irrecoverable loss. We cannot with impunity break down a single barrier which God has erected to guard His people from Satan's power." *Testimonies*, vol. 5, 199.

We are not justified in looking beyond the most widely accepted understandings of the sciences of anatomy, physiology, biochemistry, and so on, to treatment methods with other explanations of how the body is constructed and how it functions in health and disease. Neither are we justified in the use of methodologies which are not widely acknowledged to work in obedience with the natural laws of the Creator. We have more than enough to keep us busy in the use of the remedies for which we have a clear "Thus saith the Lord." It is not safe to trust in health care providers who have not the fear of God and whose practices are contrary to the laws of life or natural law:

"It is not safe to trust to physicians who have not the fear of God before them. Without the influence of divine grace the hearts of men are 'deceitful above all things, and desperately wicked.' Jeremiah 17:9. Self-aggrandizement is their aim. Under the cover of the medical profession what iniquities have been concealed, what delusions supported! The physician may claim to possess great wisdom and marvelous skill, when his character is abandoned and his practice contrary to the laws of life." Ibid., 194.

When we tamper with spiritualism or hypnosis, in any of their many forms, we lose control of our will at great peril to our eternal well-being:

"In this degenerate age Satan holds control over mortals who depart from the right, and venture upon his ground. He exercises his power upon such in an alarming manner. . . . They do not mean to enter deep into this work, but such know not what they are doing. They are venturing on the devil's ground, and are tempting him to control them. This powerful destroyer considers such his lawful prey, and will exercise his power upon them, and that against their will. When they wish to control themselves they cannot. They yielded their mind to Satan and he holds them captive, and he will not release his claims. No power can deliver the ensnared soul but the power of God, in answer to the earnest prayers of his faithful followers." *Review and Herald*, February 18, 1862.

There may be no apparent harm from using the methods promoted by Satan, but they have yet to show their full colors for the great controversy is not over:

"And while those who are devoted to these sciences laud them to the heavens because of the great and good works which they affirm are wrought by them, they little know what a power for evil they are cherishing; but it is a power which will yet work with all signs and lying wonders—with all deceivableness of unrighteousness. Mark the influence of these sciences, dear reader, for the conflict between Christ and Satan is not yet ended." *Selected Messages*, book 2, 351–352.

Yes, indeed, Satan has come down as a roaring lion seeking whom he may devour. He comes with all subtleness to deceive, if it were possible, the very elect. His agents claim that their methods work through the inherent powers of the mind, the energy currents of the body, or through energy fields or magnetism. We need to avoid all such methods, for they are very likely a mixture of truth and error—a modern-day tree of knowledge of good and evil—and they do not work, or *possibly* do not work, in part or in whole, by obedience to natural law. Thus, they are likely to be a "miracle" of Satan by which he is casting his spell upon the soul as well as the body.

Satan approaches us in a hidden manner. He works marvelously upon the bodies of those who tend to do his bidding. He works especially to deceive, if possible, the very elect:

"Satan is preparing his deceptions, that in his last campaign against the people of God they may not understand that it is he. 2 Corinthians 11:14: 'And no marvel; for Satan himself is transformed into an angel of light.'. . . He is too cunning to come openly, boldly, with his temptations;

for then the drowsy energies of the Christian would arouse, and he would rely upon the strong and mighty Deliverer. But he comes in unperceived, and works in disguise through the children of disobedience who profess godliness.

"Satan will go to the extent of his power to harass, tempt, and mislead God's people. . . . In a marvelous manner will he affect the bodies of those who are naturally inclined to do his bidding." *Testimonies*, vol. 1, 341–342.

A False Latter Rain

We are warned that just preceding the loud cry, a spurious revival promoting doctrinal error will come in among us:

"It is Satan's object now to get up new theories to divert the mind from the true work and genuine message for this time. He stirs up minds to give false interpretation of Scripture, a spurious loud cry, that the real message may not have its effect when it does come. This is one of the greatest evidences that the loud cry will soon be heard and the earth will be lightened with the glory of God." *Selected Messages*, book 3, 410.

Those among us who apostatize will use hypnotism to mislead others:

"The time has come when even in the church and in our institutions, some will depart from the faith, giving heed to seducing spirits and doctrines of devils. . . . Let us bear a plain, clear testimony right to the point, that hypnotism is being used by those who have departed from the faith, and that we are not to link up with them. Through those who depart from the faith, the power of the enemy will be exercised to lead others astray." Ibid., 411–412.

In the end-time, apostate believers will use the miracle-working power of the devil to attempt to deceive us with healings not based on natural law:

"Those who look for miracles as a sign of divine guidance are in grave danger of deception. It is stated in the Word that the enemy will work through his agents who have departed from the faith, and they will seemingly work miracles, even to the bringing down of fire out of heaven in the sight of men. By means of 'lying wonders' Satan would deceive, if possible, the very elect." Ibid., 408–409.

We are warned that those who are not living in harmony with the natural laws of health reform will interpret Satan's snares as being the providence of God:

"The fear of the Lord is the beginning of wisdom. Those who overcome as Christ overcame will need to constantly guard themselves against the temptations of Satan. The appetite and passions should be restricted and under the control of enlightened conscience, that the intellect may be unimpaired, the perceptive powers clear, so that the workings of Satan and his snares may not be interpreted to be the providence of God." *Testimonies*, vol. 3, 491.

There must be no spiritual stupidity. We need to keep ourselves clear from all practices that may be using hypnotism and/or the electric currents of Satan. Once we yield ourselves to the methods of Satan, we are increasingly susceptible to his power. Only through a knowledge of and surrender to every truth of God, as written in Inspiration and in nature, will we be protected from the miracle-working power of Satan and his agents. It is the prayer of this author that each one of us will be protected from the deceptive "miracles" of Satan as he works with all cunning and deceivableness in the area of health care and false doctrines to bring Seventh-day Adventists, as well as all Christians, to the test.

We need to keep in mind that the overriding purpose of the great controversy between Christ and Satan is to vindicate the laws of God and thus His character and government. In this end-of-time, Seventh-day Adventists have been given the special task of giving to every person on earth the call of the three angels' messages to give honor and glory to the Creator through an obedience to His natural laws as well as to His moral laws. For this purpose our generation has a wealth of knowledge regarding health reform as well as the moral truths found in the Bible. We must not be found to be cooperating with Satan in his tragic and deadly attempts to portray God's laws—and thus His character and government—as being unjust, as incapable of being obeyed and honored, and thus, as unnecessary. May the Lord help each one of us to cast our vote on the side of truth and righteousness is my prayer. ❏